MW00983893

CASE
STUDIES IN
COMMUNITY
HEALTH

CASE STUDIES IN COMMUNITY HEALTH

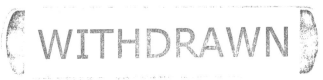

Jo Fairbanks
Judith Candelaria

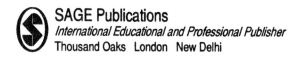

SAGE Publications
International Educational and Professional Publisher
Thousand Oaks   London   New Delhi

For information:

SAGE Publications, Inc.
2455 Teller Road
Thousand Oaks, California 91320
E-mail: order@sagepub.com

SAGE Publications Ltd.
6 Bonhill Street
London EC2A 4PU
United Kingdom

SAGE Publications India Pvt. Ltd.
M-32 Market
Greater Kailash I
New Delhi 110 048 India

Printed in the United States of America

Library of Congress Cataloging-in-Publication Data

Fairbanks, Jo.
    Case studies in community health / by Jo Fairbanks and
Judith Candelaria.
        p. cm.
    ISBN 0-7619-1405-6 (pbk.: acid-free paper)
    1. Public health—Problems, exercises, etc. 2. Public health—
Case studies. I. Candelaria, Judith. II. Title.
RA430.F34   1998
614.4—dc21   98-8878

This book is printed on acid-free paper.

98 99 00 01 02 03 04 05 8 7 6 5 4 3 2 1

Acquiring Editor:	Dan Ruth
Editorial Assistant:	Anna Howland
Production Editor:	Sherrise M. Purdum
Production Assistant:	Denise Santoyo
Typesetter/Designer:	Christina M. Hill
Print Buyer:	Anna Chin

Contents

Part III: Health Program Planning

Introduction

———— ⌒⌇⌒ ————

This book, *Case Studies in Community Health*, is written for students in public and community health courses. The purpose of the book is to help students apply critical thinking and problem-solving skills to real-life situations in public health settings. Public health practice occurs in a social context and is subject to all the complexities of a social environment. The case study approach to learning allows students to transfer knowledge and gain insight into real public and community health issues.

What is a case study? A case study typically is a description of a situation that requires some form of exploration and decision making by the student. Case studies can be from one paragraph to many pages in length. In *Case Studies in Community Health*, many of the cases are based on actual events experienced by the authors. The names of the people and the dialogue in the cases are fictional.

The book is organized into three parts: Epidemiology, Public Health Administration, and Health Program Planning. The first case study in Part I provides students with an understanding of the basic language of epidemiology. The other case studies in this part allow students to apply their knowledge of epidemiology to three very different settings.

The case studies in Part II examine the regulatory roles and administrative responsibilities of public health agencies. Through these case studies, the students will apply their knowledge of leadership and communication skills to problem solving in complex and diverse situations. Finally, this part closes with a case study on managed care and the role of public health.

Part III places the students in a variety of community practice settings for the purpose of planning health programs. Students will apply the planning process to a variety of populations in both rural and urban areas. The last case study in the book provides the students with an opportunity to develop an evaluation for the health program plan developed in a previous case.

Students may or may not have an opportunity to read the case before class. Spontaneity often improves and enlivens the discussion in class. There is no one right answer to any of the situations.

Students do have the responsibility to actively participate by applying knowledge, reason, and creativity to the discussion of the case study. Active participation includes speaking out as well as listening to others. There should be ongoing feedback between students, because it is this interaction that promotes learning.

> An Instructors Manual is available to accompany these case studies. It is highly recommended that instructors familiarize themselves with problem-based learning technques before using these cases in the classroom.

Part I

Epidemiology

Case Study #1

Basic Terms in Epidemiology

⎯⎯⎯⎯⎯⎯⎯⎯⎯⎯⎯ ৵৶ ⎯⎯⎯⎯⎯⎯⎯⎯⎯⎯⎯

Learning Objectives

At the conclusion of this case, students will be able to

1. Define and describe the most common rates used in epidemiology
2. Understand the sources of data for epidemiology
3. Describe the meaning of determinants for disease
4. Define and discuss the role of risk factors
5. Describe what data are needed to compare disease rates accurately

Y ou have just been hired as a summer intern for the Bureau of Vital Statistics in the Department of Health and Environment in your city. You are contemplating a career in this area but admit that you know little about vital statistics. The staff there is looking forward to having an intern, and they have said that you should not worry, that they will train you. You feel that this is a wonderful opportunity to learn about epidemiology and get paid for it.

This morning, your first day on the job, is the usual weekly staff meeting. Everyone gathers in the conference room. You are introduced. Everyone seems willing to help you learn, and, in fact, Bill, one of the field epidemiologists, is going on a fact-finding mission today. He invites you to come along. It seems the people of Jonstown, a nearby community, are very concerned about their health. They feel that they have far higher rates of cancer than do the other areas of the state. Bill is going to the community to talk to some of the people who have called a town meeting to discuss the issue.

You and Bill discuss the situation as you travel. Jonstown has a paper mill on the outskirts of town, as well as a large landfill. Although the landfill is no longer actively used, no one knows if it holds extremely toxic materials. The paper mill waste was buried there over the years, and the fumes from the mill are often heavy in town. People feel that there is an unusually high incidence of cancer. In response to your inquiry about his job, Bill asks you some questions:

> **What is epidemiology? What are the most common activities in which an epidemiologist would be engaged? What is an incidence rate?**

Bill tells you about his job. He acts as a resource for the state to assist in tracking disease and injuries. He helps identify determinants, the factors that are contributing to the health problem. There are many factors that can affect the incidence of cancer, such as host suscepti-bility, behavior, and the exposure to carcinogens. The environment can play a large role in cancer. Some chemicals increase the risk for cancer. You also understand that no real investigation has been done to substantiate the community's rates of illness.

> **Discuss determinants for disease. What is meant by the term? What are risk factors? What are some possible determinants or risk factors for cancer? Be sure to include host and environmental factors.**

The meeting is very interesting. It seems almost everyone in the community knows someone or has a family member who has had cancer. They want the Bureau to do research in the community to discover what could be causing it. They believe that another nearby community, Clarksville, which does not have as much environmental pollution, also does not have as much cancer.

Make a list of the basic information that is needed to begin an investigation. How do you go about getting the information?

Bill asks you to participate in this project. You call the American Cancer Society and learn that in the United States, there were approximately 1.4 million new cases of cancer diagnosed in 1997, excluding basal cell and squamous cell skin cancers. Bill wants cancer rates for the two towns that include mortality, incidence, and prevalence. Your state has a cancer registry that records patient cancer information, such as location of the patient and type and stage of cancer. You also have census data plus the resources of the Bureau, which collects morbidity and mortality data.

Discuss mortality and morbidity rates. What are they? What is the difference between incidence and prevalence rates? What does the census record? Why do we need to have this information? Rates must make sense. Discuss the numerator and the denominator for incidence rates and analyze what is needed for them.

The registry provides information on the number of patients diagnosed with cancer. You learn that the most common cancers have an unknown etiology. Census tract data are available for Jonstown and Clarksville. The Bureau collects health-related data by county, and it is not easy to get specific information on a town. You are going to have to piece together the information so that it becomes meaningful.

An important part of epidemiology is surveillance and monitoring. What information do these activities provide? Why is this important to public health? What are some of the sources of data for surveillance of disease? How are incidence, prevalence, and mortality rates derived?

Through all of your sources, you eventually discover that there actually are more diagnosed cases of cancer in Jonstown than in Clarksville. The crude mortality rate from carcinoma is also higher. Nearly 30% of deaths last year in Jonstown were due to cancer, compared to 20% for the state.

> **What is meant by a crude rate? What could be affecting the rates? Remember, you have only the number of diagnosed patients and a higher crude mortality rate than Clarksville.**

You are beginning to believe the people of Jonstown that there is more cancer in their community. You report your information to Bill. He tells you that you need much more information before drawing a conclusion.

> **What else is needed?**

You try to integrate the census information with the health statistics. Jonstown has 25,000 people, whereas Clarksville has 15,000. You had not realized the large difference in population. Of course there would be more dignosed cases of cancer in Jonstown. To understand the disease information, you need to calculate the rates so that comparisons can be made.

> **How do rates allow us to make comparisons? What comparisons do you want to make?**

You find that the most common cancer for both sexes in Jonstown is lung cancer, followed by cancer of the breast for females. Jonstown also has very high rates of prostate cancer.

> **Is this unusual? What might be affecting the rates?**

You learn through the census data that Jonstown has a very high percentage of retired people. It is a town that seems to appeal to older people, and more seem to be moving there every year. Clarksville, on the other hand, has a young population and a high birth rate.

How could this affect the rates of cancer? How do crude rates differ from age-adjusted rates? Which one will give you more accurate data for comparison?

The Bureau has completed a survey of people employed at the paper mill. It seems that employees are not experiencing rates of cancer that are higher than the rates for the United States.

What do you know about the development and the determinants of cancer that could affect whether employees would have the disease?

You know that cancer can take a long time to develop, so it may not be affecting the current workers. You conduct a phone interview with a sample of former employees. Their rate of cancer was not unusual when compared to national age-specific rates.

The people of Jonstown are right. There are more cancer diagnoses and cancer-related deaths in their community than in Clarksville. Good epidemiology, however, separates facts from fiction and makes disease rates meaningful.

Case Study #2

Cholera in London, 1850

꧁꧂

Learning Objectives

At the conclusion of this case, students will be able to

1. Describe the role of multiple determinants of a disease
2. Form hypotheses about disease causation

This is a case study that is based on an actual event. It is an illustration of the early application of the emerging principles of epidemiology. John Snow's investigation of cholera is available in its entirety in *Snow on Cholera*, New York: The Commonwealth Fund, on the Mode of Communication of Cholera (1936).

Today, we know that cholera is an acute diarrheal disease caused by an enterotoxin produced by Vibrio cholerae bacteria. The incubation period is from 1 to 6 days, but generally 2 to 3 days. Cholera causes severe dehydration, and, if not treated, has a 50% fatality rate. In the time of John Snow, bacteria as agents for disease were unknown.

Your name is John Snow. You were born in 1813, and you are living in London, England. It is 1849, and there is another outbreak of cholera in the city. You are a physician, a well-known anesthesiologist, and you are very interested in finding out how cholera is spread.

Your colleagues believe that cholera (and other disease) is caused by poison carried in the air that results from decaying matter. You have written in your journal, ". . . a view having a certain number of advocates is that cholera depends on an unknown something in the atmosphere which becomes localized, and has its effects increased by the gases given off from decomposing animal and vegetable matters." Perhaps the best attempt at explaining the disease so far was that it was communicated by effluvia given off from the patient into the surrounding air and inhaled by others into the lungs.

You disagree with your colleagues, but you have yet to prove your theory that cholera is spread by person-to-person contact. Your experience tells you that the disease can be spread from the sick to the healthy. You have many examples of this, and you write:

> A man came from Hull [where cholera was prevailing], by trade a
> painter; his name and age unknown. He lodged at the house of
> Samuel Wride at Pocklington, was attacked on his arrival on the
> 8th of September, and died on the 9th. Samuel Wride was attacked
> himself on the 11th and died shortly afterwards.

You believe that cholera commences with an affection of the alimentary canal, and you write ". . . it follows that the morbid material producing cholera must be introduced into the alimentary canal, must, in fact, be swallowed."

You also know that not everyone attending a sick person gets sick themselves, and that some people get sick even when they are not around others who are. You believe that cleanliness affects the spread of the disease, and that people attending the sick become soiled with the cholera evacuations. The disease is worse among working-class people, you think, because unless these people are scrupulously clean in their habits,

> they must accidentally swallow some of the excretion, and leave
> some on the food they prepare, which has to be eaten by the rest of

the family, who often have to take their meals in the sick room. . . .
When, on the other hand, cholera is introduced into the better
kinds of houses . . . it hardly ever spreads from one member of the
family to another. The constant use of the hand-basin and towel,
and the fact that the apartments for cooking and eating being
distinct from the sick room, are the cause of this.

**What is known so far about the disease? Think of what London
must have been like in the 1800s. How would this influence
disease theory? Why weren't physicians getting cholera if they
were treating the sick? What were the sanitary conditions like?
How do you think people got their drinking water?**

You write:

The most terrible outbreak of cholera which ever occurred in this
kingdom, is probably that which took place in Broad Street . . . a
few weeks ago. . . . There were upwards of 500 fatal attacks of
cholera in ten days. . . . On proceeding to the spot, I found that
nearly all the deaths had taken place within a short distance of the
pump (source of water). There were only 10 deaths in houses
situated nearer to another street pump. In five of these cases, the
families of the deceased informed me that they always went to the
pump in Broad Street, as they preferred the water to that which was
nearer.

**What hypothesis are you beginning to form about the spread of
cholera? How can you begin to verify your hypothesis?**

A friend who lives near Broad Street tells you that the water often
has an offensive smell. You begin to suspect that impurities in the
water are causing cholera. You have the pump handle removed and the
outbreak ends.

The water companies that provide water to the neighborhoods
pump the water from the Thames river. You are convinced that the
location of the water works near areas in the river contaminated by
sewage are the source of the problem. One of the companies, Lambeth,
has recently changed the location of their water works to an area free
from the sewage of London. The other, Southwark and Vauxhall,
remains in its previous location, pumping suspicious water.

What do you need to know to test your theory?

When cholera returns to London in July of 1854, you are ready to test your theory. You ask the General Register Office to supply you with the names of people dying of cholera in neighborhoods where the water is supplied by these two different companies.

What are you going to do? What might be obstacles to your investigation?

Here is what you eventually found:

Company	Number of Houses	Deaths	Rates in 10,000
Southwark & Vauxhall Co.	40,046	1,263	315
Lambeth Co.	26,107	98	37
Rest of London	256,423	1,422	55

What conclusions can be drawn? How might other deaths occur in the houses supplied by Lambeth?

Case Study #3

The Hantavirus Outbreak

Learning Objectives

At the conclusion of this case, students will be able to

1. Identify questions to ask when confronted with a disease outbreak of unknown cause
2. List the people and agencies to contact when a suspected outbreak occurs
3. Define and give examples of agent, vector, and host
4. Define surveillance and list three surveillance systems

You are an epidemiologist for the New Mexico Department of Health. It is late spring, 1993. Just as you are leaving for lunch, the telephone rings. The caller is the medical investigator from the area in northwestern New Mexico where four state boundaries come together, known as the Four Corners area. He has an incredible story to tell you.

"Hello, my name is Richard Jones. This morning I was called to the hospital to perform an autopsy on an athletic, 19-year-old Navajo male who died suddenly of unexplained causes. His illness was characterized by abrupt onset of fever, muscle aches, headache, and cough, rapidly progressing to respiratory failure. His chest X ray showed unexplained bilateral pulmonary interstitial infiltrates. He died within 5 hours of admission, drowning in his own fluids. Speaking to his family later in the hall, I learned that the young man, Tom, had collapsed on the way to a funeral. The funeral was for Tom's girlfriend, who had died 5 days earlier of the same symptoms. Tests for plague and other bacterial and viral pathogens are negative so far. I think we have an unknown, deadly disease here that leads very quickly to death."

> **Two people are dead from unknown causes. What is going through your mind? What information do you need to ask the medical investigator to obtain in order to start your investigation? Discuss the meaning of surveillance and possible sources of additional information about disease occurrence.**

You ask Dr. Jones to review all of his autopsy reports for any unexplained deaths due to respiratory failure in young and previously healthy people. In addition, you ask him to contact physicians in the Four Corners area about similar cases they may have seen over the past year or so. You vaguely remember your colleagues discussing some cases that had followed a similar course and were reported by the Indian Health Services. In an outbreak with a known cause, you would step up laboratory reporting; in this case, however, the agent is unknown.

The next day, Dr. Jones calls with chilling news. One physician in the Four Corners area remembered a similar case 6 months ago; the patient died. He had gone through his medical records and the county's death certificates and tentatively identified three more cases.

> **Who else needs to know right away? What other agencies need to be informed?**

You contact the health departments in Arizona, Colorado, and Utah, and, later, a review of their records indicates 24 possible cases with onset of illness dating from December 1992. Seventeen of these cases resided in New Mexico. Two more suspicious cases are called in to the health department. You are getting very worried.

The 17 New Mexico deaths of unknown causes since 1992 do not represent a lot of fatalities; why worry? What is the next step?

Extensive interviews with family and friends of the victims reveal that most were Navajo from rural areas. They were active young people who enjoyed outdoor activities. In addition, you learn that the brother and sister-in-law of Tom had recently moved into his house with their infant son. They both became very ill but survived. Their infant remained well. You review all known cases and learn that none is younger than twelve.

List what you know so far about this disease.

Nineteen days have passed since the first call from Dr. Jones. The pathogen has not been identified. There are still no answers; in fact, there are far more questions than answers. Why is this disease only of young, active, healthy people who live in the Four Corners area? Is it transmitted from person to person? What protective measures can be taken?

The University of New Mexico Hospital and Medical School staff are trying to identify the pathogen. By the 17th of May, 16 new cases have been reported, and University Hospital is caring for them. More help is needed. A team of scientists from the Centers for Disease Control arrives 2 days after the Memorial Day weekend. The media finds out and besieges the hospital and your office.

What are the issues regarding disclosure of this disease? It is the beginning of tourist season in New Mexico. What is the public's "right to know"?

The newspapers begin calling it the "Navajo Disease." The stereotyping results in angry responses and delays the investigation. It is harder to get tribal members to talk to you. Tourism begins to decline. The media reports everything, including rumors, and your phone is ringing constantly. Political leaders are calling for answers immediately. Through the interviews, you learn that the cases seem to be associated with wood piles and garbage cans near the houses, outdoor activities, and airing out buildings that had evidence of mice.

> **Using an epidemiological model, what hypothesis are you beginning to form? Examine what you know by describing the characteristics of time, place, and person in this outbreak.**

Finally, some answers! Clinical and autopsy specimens analyzed by the CDC laboratories find rising titers of antibodies to hantaviruses. You know that these viruses are responsible for several types of hemorrhagic fevers in the world. The CDC reports that this strain of hantavirus is unknown. You know that rodents usually carry the virus.

> **What do you do now?**

Humans are thought to be at risk for hantavirus infection after exposure to rodent excreta, either through the aerosol route or direct inoculation. Trapping and testing rodents in the Four Corners area reveals the deer mouse as the likely source of the hantavirus.

> **Identify and discuss the "agent," the "vector," and the "host." You wonder why the disease has remained unnoticed until now. What are some possible determinants of the disease? What might be going on environmentally that could affect this epidemic?**

In the spring of 1993, an unusual chain of events occurred. An environmentalist noticed an increase in the numbers of deer mice, thus the probability of increased exposure to the rodent. You also learn from a field biologist that due to a very wet year in 1992, the piñon pine provided an abundance of nuts, which are the primary food for deer mice. This plentiful food source resulted in an increase in the population of the rodent.

> **What interventions are possible to end this outbreak? What educational measures need to be undertaken? Who are the key**

players in this outbreak? What agencies need to cooperate? What obstacles would be expected? How do you communicate information about the outbreak to the public and private sectors?

This case is based on an actual outbreak of hantavirus in New Mexico. Hantaviruses cause diseases characterized by abrupt onset of fever, prostration, backache, headache, abdominal pain, and vomiting, often followed by renal or pulmonary failure. They are responsible for different diseases in different parts of the world. Field rodents are the reservoir, and it is presumed that infections in humans occur when tiny droplets of infected rodent excreta are inhaled. Preventive measures include minimizing exposure to rodents and their excreta and spraying rodent-contaminated areas with a disinfectant prior to cleaning. This particular virus does not seem to be transmitted from person to person. The incubation period ranges from 5 to 42 days. There is no known cure for the disease. The outbreak was over by the fall of 1993.

What can be done to prevent future disease?

Case Study #4

Focus on Violence

==

Learning Objectives

At the conclusion of this case, students will be able to

1. Discuss violence from an epidemiologic perspective
2. Identify the data required to analyze violence in a community
3. List sources of violence data

==

Homicide, suicide, child and elder abuse, battered women, sexual assault, and domestic violence—these issues confront you daily through newspapers and television.

You are the program developer for the community health center in which you work. Your responsibilities include assessing community needs, building community and agency coalitions around those needs, developing strategies and programs to address the issues, and writing grants to secure funding.

Your community health center provides primary health care to 10,000 inner-city residents in a metropolitan area. The health center also provides outpatient mental health care and social services.

Last week, an enraged young man waving his fists came screaming into the health center. "Where is Mary?" he yelled. "I told her not to leave the house." Mary was cowering in the social worker's office. She had come in to see the nurse practitioner for birth control pills and was referred to the social worker because of suspicious bruises on her face and body.

The health center had in place a procedure for handling potentially violent situations. A panic button behind the receptionist's desk brought the police within minutes. However, staff were still very nervous because they were becoming increasingly aware of abused women and children in the health center. After the police were called and Mary transported to a shelter for battered women, the staff debriefed the incident.

The staff wondered how extensive the violence is in the community. You decide that this is an area for further exploration.

> **Discuss the different types of violence. Why are you concerned about violence? What is the relationship of violence to health? How are medical care costs affected? Why is it a public health issue? What do you know about the determinants and contributing factors of violence? Is this an area of concern to the whole community? What role does the health center have in violence prevention?**

As you leaf through your mail, you come across a brochure from the university's continuing education department. They are offering an educational activity titled "The Roots of Violence in America." Noting that continuing education credit is offered for nurses, doctors, social workers, and health educators, you register a multidisciplinary group (including yourself) from the health center to attend this educational activity.

At the conference, you learn that youth violence has risen dramatically. There are more than one million people in state prisons—most of them poor, young, minority males. Forty-six percent of them are in prison for crimes of violence. The United States experiences an average of 21,000 murders each year. You are told that it is not like this everywhere. In 1990, more than 10,000 people in the United States were killed by handguns, as compared with 87 in Japan and 22 in Great Britain.

Before attending this conference, you believed that violence was a random act that occurred to someone else. Violence was perceived to be an accident, not something that could be prevented. Now you know that most violence occurs between people who know each other. A woman in the United States is more likely to be injured, raped, or killed by a boyfriend, spouse, or ex-husband than by a stranger. Young children are more likely to be sexually assaulted by their father, stepfather, mother's boyfriend, or other trusted friend or relative. Most elder abuse occurs by friends or relatives who are the caregivers in their own homes. You also learned that there is a direct relationship between violence and substance abuse. And, if you keep a gun in the house, you or a family member are more likely to be killed or injured by it than an intruder.

What are other contributing factors to violence? Discuss what data you want to collect in order to assess the problem of violence in your community.

You are beginning to understand the relationship of all the various forms of violence and the factors contributing to it. Abused children become abusing adults. Thirty percent of murdered women are killed by their male partners and have a prior history of being battered. Although violence occurs at all socioeconomic levels, the poor bear a disproportionate burden of violent behaviors. The number of children living in poverty has increased markedly over the past 5 years. The high school dropout rate also is high. The media messages are especially influential on the young. The average child sees 16,000 murders on TV by the time he or she leaves high school. The alteration of family and community structure because of mobility, single-parent families, and families in which both parents work creates stress and an erosion of support factors.

Identify the federal and state agencies that may have data on
violence. Where can you go to get violence data that reflect your
community?

First, you go to the Department of Public Safety to get crime
statistics. You learn that the homicide rate per 100,000 population is
13 in your community, as compared to 11 for the state and 10 for the
nation. The police department's crime report shows that there are
1,000 assaults and 70 rapes per 100,000 population. This is higher
than the state rates of 700 and 60, respectively. The nation's rates are
even less—400 and 40. Interviews with the Office of the Medical
Investigator and the Rape Crisis Center confirm your fears. Homicide
and personal assault are major problems in your community.

You go to the library to review census data. There, you find that the
per capita income is lower, and the percentage of families headed by a
single parent is higher, than for the rest of your state. You also go to
the State Department of Education and learn that the dropout rate in
the school district in which your health center is located is high.

Child and elder abuse are reportable to the child and adult protective
service division in the human services department in your county. You
learn there that child abuse investigations have doubled in the past 3
years. The child abuse rate is 70 per 1,000 children in the community
as compared to 50 in the state and 45 in the nation. Adult abuse
investigations also are increasing, from 520 three years ago to 986 last
year.

Create a table comparing your community's violence data with
state and national data. What are the implications of these
statistics? What else do you need to know to describe the
violence problem in your community? What agencies can you
contact for additional information? What can be done? Develop
a cause-and-effect model of violence relevant to this community.

Violence is more readily addressed when approached from an
epidemiologic perspective. Violent acts are seldom random. Collection
of data from the community on what, when, where, how, and who can
lead to specific interventions to reduce violence. Building partnerships
with other interested organizations in the community will strengthen
the efforts toward violence prevention.

Part II

Public Health Administration

Case Study #5

Why Regulate?

———————————— ✿ ————————————

===

Learning Objectives

At the conclusion of this case, students will be able to

1. Understand the mission, substance, and organization of public health
2. Understand the purpose of regulation in the protection of the public's health
3. Become more familiar with the multilevel agencies and organizations engaged in public health activities

===

The Institute of Medicine defines the *mission* of public health as the fulfillment of society's interest in ensuring the conditions in which people can be healthy. The *substance* of public health is defined as organized community efforts aimed at the prevention of disease and promotion of health. It links many disciplines and rests upon the scientific core of epidemiology. The organizational framework of public health encompasses both activities undertaken within the formal structure of government and the associated efforts of private and voluntary organizations and individuals (Institute of Medicine, 1988, pp. 40-42).

There are federal, state, and local public health agencies. There are governmental, not-for-profit, and private organizations engaged in public health activities. Public health efforts are being carried out at all levels all around us. Public health activities began in ancient history with early attempts to protect the population from disease. These protection initiatives continue today, but the focus of public health has broadened.

You were reading the newspaper a few days ago and noticed that several people had recently been admitted to the hospital in your community for gastrointestinal symptoms attributed to "food poisoning." On two or three occasions in your life, you suspected that you had food poisoning, but you were never sick enough to go to the hospital.

Why might this hospitalization of a few people be a public health concern?

You read later that three more people, including two children, have been hospitalized, and the paper says that the State Office of Epidemiology has started an investigation.

What's going on? What is this office, and what are they doing? Why is it important to you and your community?

Yesterday, you read that people are still getting sick, and one child has died. The hospital has discovered that the food poisoning outbreak is caused by a particular strain of *Escherichia coli* bacteria (0157:H7), but no one knows where it is coming from. You do some research and find out that *E. coli* bacteria grow in the intestine, and some strains produce a toxin that makes people very sick for a few days. Although most people recover, you learn that it is especially dangerous for the elderly and for small children. It is found in animal feces, so you wonder how it is getting into what people are eating.

> How did the hospital find out what was causing the problem?
> What do you think the investigators from the office of
> epidemiology are doing now? What would you do to find out how
> people are coming in contact with the bacteria?

Today's paper says that most of the people who have been hospital-ized have lived or worked in the north side of town. It says that a north-side restaurant is probably the source of the contaminated food, but investigators are not yet sure which one. You decide not to go out for dinner tonight.

> How could *E. coli* be getting into the restaurant's food? What
> does all this have to do with public health? If this were
> happening in your state, which agencies and organizations
> would be involved in the regulation of food? How do public
> health laws protect communities? What is regulated and why?
> Make a list of all the agencies and organizations you can think
> of that are engaged in public health activities. Include federal as
> well as state and local agencies. How many are regulatory? Why
> regulate?

Reference

Institute of Medicine. (1988). *Future of public health*. Washington, DC: Author.

Case Study #6

Meningococcal Meningitis Outbreak

—————————— ❧ ——————————

===
Learning Objectives

At the conclusion of this case, students will be able to

1. Describe the administrative responsibilities of a county health officer
2. Discuss public health law
3. List the steps involved in developing a media advocacy plan
4. List the major barriers to implementing a public health intervention
===

You are a physician practicing in Benton County. Benton County is a sparsely populated, rural county of 9,000 people in northwestern Indiana. The location of the county seat and your private practice is in Fowler. Fowler is a town of 2,500. Most of the people in Benton County have small farms.

The county commissioners asked you to be the health officer of Benton County because you are the only physician in this county. Your private practice is not very busy, and you feel you can easily handle both jobs, so you accept their offer.

What do you think are the functions and responsibilities of a county health officer?

After accepting the role of county health officer for Benton County, you learn that you have multiple responsibilities. You need to understand the health status of the population in your county. You are responsible to the community for clean air, water, food, and protection from infectious diseases. You are required to enforce public health laws around these issues. When necessary, you will also develop and support health policy that affects your community.

Three weeks into your job as county health commissioner, you hear some startling news from the mother of one of your patients. A student (and classmate of your patient) who attends Fowler Elementary School was hospitalized in Indianapolis the previous day while visiting the Capitol Building. The 8-year-old child suddenly became ill with a high fever, severe headache, and rash. "Oh no," you say out loud. "Are we going to have an outbreak of measles in our school?" The mother of your patient tells you that she heard that it was not measles but some kind of meningitis. She wonders if she should fear for her own child's health.

You are reminded of the seriousness of meningococcal meningitis, one form of bacterial meningitis. This infectious disease is characterized by a sudden onset of fever, intense headache, stiff neck, nausea and vomiting, and, frequently, a rash. Even with early diagnosis, the fatality rate is between 5% and 15%.

What information does the county health officer need to obtain? Who should she contact first? What is the role of the laboratory? What is a fatality rate?

After a few frustrating phone calls to the Children's Hospital in Indianapolis, you finally reach the child's attending physician and learn that the diagnosis has been confirmed by the laboratory as meningococcal meningitis. And, sadly, the child died of overwhelming sepsis. Your throat goes dry as you think of your own son, who also attends Fowler Elementary. You know that meningococcal disease is an extremely serious illness with a 50% fatality rate when not recognized early enough. It is characterized by early symptoms that could be misdiagnosed as the flu. Delirium and coma often follow. It is communicable through exposure to the respiratory droplets of infected people and usually has an incubation period of 3 to 4 days. Up to 10% of people may carry the meningococcal organism in their noses and throats without showing any signs of illness. Quick prophylaxis of intimate contacts with an effective antibiotic can help prevent additional cases.

What does the county health officer do now? Who is at risk for catching this disease? Who else needs to know about this? What regulations affect this disease?

Learning that the physician in Indianapolis provided antibiotics to all of the child's family, you send the public health nurse to the elementary school with a flyer to be sent home with all of the child's classmates. It describes the early signs of illness and recommends that parents come to the elementary school the next morning to pick up prescriptions for antibiotics.

Feeling that the public health nurse has everything under control at the school, you return to your office to see patients. Your first patient is a 12-year-old from the local Catholic school. He is presenting with rapid onset of fever, headache, and delirium. You send the patient immediately to the county hospital emergency room with orders that hospital personnel collect cerebral spinal fluid and blood for cultures and treat for meningococcal disease. You are concerned about his classmates, his family, and other children with whom he has played in the past few days.

Your next two patients are a husband and wife in their 50s who own a small farm 25 miles away. Their 25-year-old son brought them in to see you because they had symptoms similar to the child who died. Your examination leads you to the suspicion that they, too, have meningococcal meningitis. The son is a teacher at the elementary school.

> What is going on? List the confirmed and suspected cases. What
> might be the connections between cases?

As soon as you heard about the case in Indianapolis, you called the
state epidemiologist at the State Department of Health. Meningococcal disease is reportable to the State Department of Health. He told
you to call immediately if you learned of any other cases. You call him
again and review together the circumstances of all of the suspected
cases. By now, you have laboratory confirmation for the 12-year-old.
The state epidemiologist tells you that a telephone report just came
in about a set of 13-year-old twins who live in a small town in Benton
County and attend the Catholic school. They were diagnosed as
having meningococcal meningitis in an adjacent county.

> What is a reportable disease? Who reports what to whom, and by
> what means?

He informs you that meningococcal outbreaks are either point
source outbreaks or community outbreaks. Point source outbreaks
usually occur in an institution such as a school and spread rapidly.
Community outbreaks are when no single institution seems to be
involved, and when the outbreak is slow and protracted. Meningococcal vaccine has been shown to be effective for adults in community
outbreaks. You are puzzled. This outbreak could be either a classic
point source or community outbreak.

> Use a decision-making process to determine an intervention for
> a point source and a community outbreak of meningococcal
> meningitis.

As soon as you hang up the telephone, it rings. The caller identifies
herself as Sharon Mills from WXLW-TV. She wants to know what you
are going to do about the outbreak of this deadly disease. This is your
first encounter with the media, and your tendency is to tell her
nothing. She is persistent, and you feel threatened. As your dialogue
with her continues, you realize that she would have been less suspicious of your intentions if you had contacted her first. You make a
mental note to build relationships with all of the media reporters who
cover health issues. You could even start a health column in the local

newspaper. The media are a good resource for relaying information to the public.

As the person responsible for controlling this outbreak, list the steps you need to take to control this outbreak. What nonmedical issues will influence your decision making? What barriers do you expect in implementing a public health response to this crisis?

You are not sure whether this is a point source outbreak or a community outbreak. But new cases are occurring rapidly, and people are panicking. The county commissioners look to you for help, but they want you to reveal as little as possible to the public. You don't have enough resources or time to carefully investigate every case to identify true contacts, but you want to provide antibiotic prophylaxis to those who say they are a contact. You could immunize the entire county to stop this outbreak. This plan would cost the county more than $50,000—dollars that were not budgeted.

How are you going to proceed? It would be fear-producing, costly, and require considerable personnel to immunize the whole county. Are there less radical solutions?

Your job is to protect the population. Public health law requires that you act in the public's best interest, even when your decisions are not politically expedient. You decide to view this as a community outbreak and forge ahead.

Over the next 3 days, and using the middle school as the base of operations, you, the public health nurse, the school nurse, and a couple of staff from the State Department of Health provide antibiotic prophylaxes to those who say they are a contact. You also immunize 3,000 people in the county who heard about the mass immunization effort via word of mouth and the radio. Two weeks have passed, and there have been no new cases.

Case Study #7

Quality Leadership Process

⸎

Learning Objectives

At the conclusion of this case, students will be able to

1. Select an appropriate leadership style when managing a communicable disease outbreak that involves several jurisdictions and sectors of the community
2. Discuss the communication skills needed when facilitating a group of public health officials and private sector players who have different agendas
3. Discuss the elements required for team building

You are the supervising nurse epidemiologist for a city-county health department in a western state. The health department in which you work is responsible for public health services in a sprawling urban area of 2,500 square miles containing 1 million people. The state capitol and the state health department are located in your city.

On an unusually warm Tuesday morning in February, you get a call from the state epidemiologist, Dr. Jenkins. Dr. Jenkins says, "Bill, you won't believe what is happening! We have a problem." He is so distraught, you ask him to slow down. He tells you the following story:

"Late yesterday, I received a call from the coach of the Jefferson High School basketball team. On Saturday night, the team won the state semi-final basketball championship here in the city-county sports arena where high school basketball teams and their supporters from all over the state have been congregating since Friday night. On Monday morning, Coach Martin received several calls from his players and their parents. They were sick with fever, headache, stomach cramps, vomiting, and diarrhea. Coach Martin consulted with the team trainer, who advised him to call the state health department."

Your throat goes dry as you remember the phone message you received early this morning but had not yet returned because of your staff meeting. It was a message from the infection control nurse at City Hospital about an unusual number of visits to the emergency room over the weekend by people with the same symptoms.

What is your immediate reaction to this story? What questions do you need to ask?

Dr. Jenkins goes on to say that the illnesses have not been diagnosed, but he suspects a common source outbreak due to contaminated food or water consumed in the sports arena. You recognize that the potential for additional reports of illness is high. Thousands of people have consumed food and water in the arena over the past few days. Additional fears enter your thoughts. Teams are practicing in the arena all week. The state finals are scheduled to begin in the same arena this Friday night. Dr. Jenkins is so concerned about the potential involvement of the outbreak that he called in the Centers for Disease Control (CDC) before calling you.

As you put the telephone down, it rings again. It's a reporter from Channel 12—a major television station in the city. The reporter, who covers the City Hospital emergency room, wants to know what is going on and what you are going to do about it. She wants to come to your office over the lunch hour to do a live report for the noon news.

List the potential jurisdictions involved in this outbreak. List the segments of the private sector that have a stake in the outbreak. Analyze possible areas of conflict between jurisdictions and with the private sector when developing a public health response to this emergency.

Your city-county health officer is on vacation and has left you in charge of the public health department during her absence. You have worked as a nurse epidemiologist in communicable disease control in this health department for the past 10 years. During other outbreaks, you have worked with officials from the Centers for Disease Control and the state health department. You also are well-known and respected by the media, local hospitals, and private health care providers. Your philosophy is that public health officials closest to the problem are best equipped to develop and manage an effective public health response, with support and technical assistance from federal and state agencies. You also believe that there is a role for the private sector when developing a public health response.

As a member of the community, you are sensitive to the needs of the media and concerns of the public. The media may pressure you to cancel all practice sessions in the arena this week. The business community, on the other hand, expects you to track down the source of the problem and resolve it before they lose business. Thousands of basketball fans will be visiting the city this weekend, staying in hotels, eating at restaurants, and shopping at malls. Private sector health care providers will look to you for answers as they field questions and concerns from their patients.

Sitting down at your desk, you begin to evaluate all of the information you have so far. In your jurisdiction, you are faced with an outbreak of a serious, yet-to-be-identified disease that seems to have a common source. A number of official agencies are involved. The federal agency, because of the potential of this outbreak, wants to send its own epidemiologists into your jurisdiction. The state health department also has its responsibilities in outbreak control from a statewide perspective. As the person in charge of the city-county health department over the outbreak, you have to play a leadership role. Leadership is the means by which goals are accomplished. Immediate intervention is critical!

What leadership characteristics can be applied in this situation? What values and principles can you promote?

You realize that your office needs to provide leadership through clear and timely communication. Because you do not have all of the expertise or resources required to intervene in this outbreak, you will rely on help from other jurisdictions. Your connections with the other jurisdictions and the community will add to your effectiveness. You decide that the intervention will be a team effort.

Who needs to be involved in the decision making? How can decisions be made?

An epidemiologist from CDC arrives on Wednesday morning. You have assembled a group of people: an epidemiologist from the state health department, the CDC epidemiologist, the infection control nurse from the hospital, the director of the City Environmental Health Department, and the manager of the sports arena.

CDC wants to send a contingent of epidemiologists to the scene to take specimens and do interviews. They envision a major scientific article here. You want to set up a hotline for the public to call in so that you can gather more information and determine the cause of this outbreak. The Environmental Health Department wants to start taking water and food samples from the concession stands in the arena. They also want all public health nurses assigned to do food histories on people with symptoms. The sports arena manager does not want the media involved. The state epidemiologist just listens.

What techniques can you use for handling differing agendas from different jurisdictions? How will you build this team in order to execute an appropriate public health response in a timely way?

As the facilitator of this assembly of people, you have prepared a meeting agenda and assigned the roles of note taker and timekeeper. The group needs to stay on target, and a recording of the proceedings and decisions needs to be kept. You ask the group what else needs to be put on the agenda. The group develops ground rules for its proceedings. The ground rules are the following:

- Speak one at a time
- Participate in the discussion
- Respect everyone's opinion
- Seek to understand
- Listen

The next step in developing this team is to agree on its goals. Using a consensus-building exercise, the group agrees that the primary goal is to determine and eliminate the source of the outbreak as quickly as possible. Your job is to keep the goal in front of the team, clarify the path to the goal, and minimize obstructions. The principles the group has agreed on are the following:

- Value all opinions
- Acknowledge concerns
- Disseminate clear and timely messages to the public

With adoptions of the agenda, ground rules, goals, and principles, the group is ready to design a step-by-step intervention.

Managed Care:
What Role for Public Health?

━━━━━━━━━━━━━━━ ❦ ━━━━━━━━━━━━━━━

━━━━━━━━━━━━━━━━━━━━━━━━━━━━━━━━━━

Learning Objectives

At the conclusion of this case, students will be able to

1. Discuss the current financial concerns about health care
2. Understand the role of managed care as a cost-cutting measure
3. Identify the principles of managed care
4. List the barriers inherent in managed care
5. Discuss the role of assurance in managed care
6. Discuss the issues around the role of public health in a managed care system, including ethical considerations

━━━━━━━━━━━━━━━━━━━━━━━━━━━━━━━━━━

Y ou are a public health nurse in the Hopewell County public health office, which is in a rural community. Managed care for Medicaid clients became effective in your state 1 month ago. You are not that familiar with managed care. You understand that the rising cost of health care delivery is encouraging new strategies for cost containment. You were in a workshop recently where the discussion was about managed care. You learned that $988.5 billion dollars were spent on health care nationally in 1995. This represented 13.6% of the U.S. gross domestic product. Rising costs affect both private and public financing systems. Resources are limited, and when health care takes a growing percentage of the budget, less money is available for other programs. You learned that managed care organizations insure members and provide care through a defined network of providers. They also manage the practice of those providers. Primary care providers act as "gatekeepers," controlling the patient's access to specialty services, medical tests, and procedures; they also limit hospital stays. Patients are restricted to a provider network and certain hospitals. Managed care organizations (MCOs) often negotiate a fixed cost per member per year. This "capitated" per-member rate is paid to the providers for total care, whether the patient receives services or not. When members stay well, providers prosper; when members are very ill, the costs of that care must be borne by the provider group.

The Johnson Medical Group (JMG) was awarded the state contract for Medicaid managed care in Hopewell County. Every person eligible for Medicaid will now receive health care from providers affiliated with JMG. JMG is a managed care organization with providers all over the state. Dr. Jamison is the only provider in your town who belongs to the JMG.

> **Discuss managed care in your group. What are advantages and disadvantages to this system? How can it reduce health care expenditures? How does this affect access? How can limiting hospital stays affect patient care? What about patient satisfaction? What are the disadvantages to providers?**

It is Wednesday morning, and as you unlock the public health office door, Maria Caborelli steps in. You've known Maria for years. She received prenatal care from the public health nurse practitioner 2 years ago when she was pregnant with her first child, Timmy. She's been bringing Timmy in regularly for his immunizations. Maria looks worried. "I think I'm pregnant again," she says. A pregnancy test confirms her suspicions. By your calculations, Maria is 8 weeks pregnant.

Maria sighs in resignation, "Well, set me an appointment with that nice nurse who took care of me during my last pregnancy. She was the one who discovered I had too much sugar in my blood while I was pregnant." You know that Maria is eligible for Medicaid and will need to go to Dr. Jamison. You try to explain this to Maria, who says that she likes the nurse in the public health office better and Dr. Jamison's office is too far away. She does not have transportation. Besides, she does not want to get on Medicaid again. It's just too complicated. You explain that the health department can no longer provide prenatal or well child care. Under the new regulations, the public health office cannot receive Medicaid reimbursement for these services. Prior to Medicaid managed care, the health department successfully billed Medicaid for services provided. This helped pay for the nurse practitioner. You tell Maria that she and Timmy will not be able to receive care from the clinic any longer.

What are the choices for Maria? How can you help?

After explaining the Medicaid enrollment process to Maria, you help her call for an appointment at the Medicaid office. You learn that Medicaid pays for transportation to health care appointments. Then you give Maria Dr. Jamison's telephone number and urge her to call for her first prenatal appointment as soon as she can. She also needs to schedule an appointment for Timmy.

Three weeks later, Maria is back at the public health office crying. She has not been able to see the doctor because the nurse would not make an appointment until she got her Medicaid number. "I went to the Medicaid office like you said. At first, they told me I had to look for a job. She called it welfare reform. When I explained that I was pregnant and not feeling well, the lady at the Medicaid office told me that the rule didn't apply to pregnant women. Why couldn't she have told me that in the first place? Anyway, I filled out all the papers, got a Medicaid number, and called Dr. Jamison. His nurse said he couldn't see me for 6 weeks. I am not feeling well. I will be more than 4 months pregnant before I see the doctor. What am I going to do?"

Discuss the barriers of a capitated Medicaid managed care system in a rural community. What are the ethical considerations?

Later that day, you meet with your supervisor—the county health department manager. You explain the dilemma of Maria and others like her not gaining timely access to their designated health care provider. Maria is now 11 weeks pregnant and at high risk for gestational diabetes because of her previous history. Janet, the county health department manager, says, "We cannot compete with JMG for patients. There is no funding for us to provide direct clinical services. We are out of the service delivery business. We need to focus more on community development, broader population issues, and prevention strategies." Traditionally, public health has been the provider for patients without access to other providers. You ask Janet, "Just what is our responsibility here?"

What are the problems from Maria's point of view? What could the health department do to continue to ensure care in the community?

As you and your county health department manager discuss the issues around access and equity in a Medicaid managed care system, you decide that one designated provider in the area is not sufficient to meet the health care needs of the Medicaid population. It would be impossible for one provider to see the numbers of Medicaid patients in the area. You feel that there is a definite role for the public health clinic. Together, the two of you make an appointment with the manager of the JMG health plan to discuss a possible contract between JMG and the county health department for services Dr. Jamison is unable to provide—prenatal care, family planning, well child care. Janet insists that a fee-for-service contract would be the only acceptable way for the MCO to reimburse the public health clinic for clinical services.

What is fee for service? Why is fee for service more beneficial than a capitated fee?

You schedule a meeting with Don Torrence, the manager of JMG's health plan, the county health department manager, and yourself for next Wednesday. Armed with data on the number of Medicaid-eligible women and children in your community needing family planning, prenatal care, and well child care, you clearly demonstrate that Dr. Jamison does not have the capacity to provide care for all of these people. Don scratches his chin and exclaims, "I had no idea there were this many potential Medicaid patients. In our contract with the state, we are obligated to enroll these people into our system and provide care."

You explain to Mr. Torrence that the staff in your public health office have been providing family planning, prenatal, and well child services for many years. The primary roles of public health are to gather data about health status and health resources in the community, facilitate the development of health systems where needed in a community, address health issues affecting populations, and focus on prevention. However, when communities are unable to meet the health care needs of their service areas, the health department can and should provide those services. "How can we work together to ensure that all of these functions are accomplished?" you ask.

Over the next few weeks, the three of you develop an action plan to answer that question. Developing the plan presented many difficulties. Janet reluctantly agrees to allow your staff to provide family planning, prenatal care, and well child care to the Medicaid population unable to be seen by Dr. Jamison for a negotiated capitated fee. Mr. Torrence agrees to actively recruit another family practice physician in the area to become a member of JMG. You set up a meeting with the medical director of JMG to negotiate the incorporation of clinical preventive and health promotion standards into their protocols. Janet agrees to work with the county commissioners to schedule a town meeting so that the community can begin to address the problems of access to health care in their town.

Back at the office, you and your supervisor are very pleased with the progress that just occurred. "We will still be able to meet our mission of ensuring access to health care, developing community approaches to solving health problems, and integrating disease prevention and health promotion strategies into population-focused practice."

Part III

Health Program Planning

Case Study #9

Planning in a Social Context

Learning Objectives

At the conclusion of this case, students will be able to

1. Understand that public health planning occurs in a social environment within all the complexities of that environment
2. Discuss the role for needs assessment, including focus groups for qualitative data
3. Realize that successful planning depends on community involvement and ownership

You work as a health planner in a regional office of the Department of Health (DOH). In your state, the main offices and administration are located in the state capital, but there are also four regional offices. The regional offices house a service unit, which has a medical director and provides basic primary care in satellite offices throughout the region. Your state is very rural, and without these services, many people would not have access to primary care.

You have recently conducted a health survey in your region for the DOH. The survey results indicate diabetes rates that are the highest in the state. The survey also shows that elderly respondents did not exercise, did not avoid fat in their diet, and were overweight. Of women over 30 years of age, 50% had not had a PAP smear or a breast exam in the past 2 years. There were higher than average rates of motor vehicle accidents, and more than 70% of the population surveyed did not regularly wear seatbelts.

You realize that the survey results were based on information gathered at the DOH clinics on a small sample of patients, and you want to know more. At the next staff meeting, you report the survey results and say that you think the department should do something about these health concerns. The consensus is that the community needs to get involved.

> **What is meant by community? Establish demographics for an imagined community, and use this community for the rest of the case study. Who lives here? Elderly? Poor? Ethnic mix? What are the cultural differences in the people in your area? After you have developed your community, decide which factors might be influencing the survey results.**

You decide to organize six focus groups to ascertain community health concerns.

> **How do you get started? Who should be included? What is meant by "inside and outside" solutions? You live here, and the DOH is here. Where do you fit in? Organize your groups based on the community's demographics and characteristics. To whom do you talk? How can you make sure that you have "real community" representation?**

> **Remember: Focus groups should be organized around a single question. What question will you want your groups to answer?**

At the end of the meetings, people stay and talk. You are surprised that the results are so similar. The community does not separate their health concerns from other concerns. They see their problems as interrelated. They are worried about high rates of unemployment and drug and alcohol use among young people. They see them dying from drinking and driving. They are afraid that family values are eroding, and their kids are out of control. They do not know their neighbors anymore. The older people do not come outside and socialize much anymore.

Summarize the results of your focus groups. What is the next step? How can the community come together around these issues? How do you prioritize? Begin to formulate a health plan. What is the primary concern you are going to undertake? What are the behavioral determinants? What is the social environment's role as a contributor? What are other factors influencing the problem? List determinants from all levels, including host, agent, and environment. What would an intervention plan look like at this point? How can the schools and neighborhoods be involved? What are major barriers that may be encountered?

Case Study #10

Closure of a
Planned Parenthood Clinic

꿎

Learning Objectives

At the conclusion of this case, students will be able to

1. Assess the impact of the closing of a major health care provider in a community
2. Discuss the information required to do a family planning needs assessment in a community
3. Describe the strategies used to meet the family planning needs in a community
4. Apply the core public health functions to health planning

Y ou are the county health manager in a southwestern state that borders Mexico. Currently, 150,000 people live in the county; 37,000 of them are women of childbearing age. The population is expected to double in 15 years. With a per capita income of just over

$13,000 per year, more than 20% of the population is below the poverty level. The county seat is a midsized city of 110,000. Surrounding the city are farmland, river frontage, desert, and rocky mountains.

Despite the rapidly exploding population, the increase in numbers of legal and illegal immigrants from Mexico, and the low socio-economic status of the population, you are feeling optimistic about the availability and quality of health care providers in the county. Health care facilities in the county that provide services to the poor include a hospital-based clinic for women and children, two community health centers, two Planned Parenthood clinics, and several public health clinics. There is even a health council in the community that is composed of health and social service professionals as well as consumers. People value health and health care here.

Just as you prepare to go into the weekly meeting with your management team, the telephone rings. It is Jane Wilson, the state family planning program manager. "John," she says. "We have a problem. The Planned Parenthood clinics in your county are closing down due to lack of funding. We've been working with them for a year and a half without success to help them comply with state and federal family planning contracting requirements. As a result, we can no longer legally support their activities. We are withdrawing their state and federal financial support."

> **What impact will the closing of Planned Parenthood have on this community? What are the short- and long-term consequences of limiting access to family planning services?**

You open up the management team meeting with a discussion of the problem. Doris, the nursing manager, had some statistics to share. "The birth rate in this county of 20.1 is higher than the nation. Nineteen percent of all the births are to teens and 40% to single mothers. Twenty to 40% of all pregnancies in the county are unintended."

> **What have you assessed so far? Describe the population affected. What other resources for family planning might be available?**

Others on the management team begin a lively dialogue. "We haven't had to provide family planning services before. How can we gear up to do this with our current resources?" "Should we step in and provide services? Or, can we ensure that other providers will fill this gap?" "How can continuity of care occur when services are abruptly interrupted?"

Just as you were trying to restore order in the room, there was a timid knock on the door as it slowly opened. It was your secretary. "I need some help. The telephones are ringing off the wall at our public health offices. Apparently, there is a sign on the Planned Parenthood clinic door that it has gone out of business and that the building is sold. Patients are calling us for assistance."

What do you need to know to develop a plan of action? List the steps to take in conducting an assessment of community needs and resources around family planning. Discuss the role of the community in public health practice.

After the office manager left the management meeting to see how she could help staff handle the phones, the discussion continued. Dr. Jim Franks, the county health officer, reviewed in his mind the current clinic assignments of the nurse practitioners and physician assistants he supervised. He knew there were other family planning providers in the county, but they either had waiting lists or refused to see uninsured people. Out loud, he said, "Somehow, we have to find a way to fill the gap." Finally, Doris spoke again, "John, we will need space, equipment, supplies, pharmaceuticals, and trained staff to provide family planning services. We will need the clinical records from the Planned Parenthood clinics in order to provide appropriate services."

Soon, it was painfully clear to you that many issues needed to be resolved. He knew they had to come up with a workable plan and fast.

Who are the key players around family planning issues in the community? What agendas will you expect from the key players? How would you bring them to the table?

Before the meeting was adjourned, assignments were made, and Dr. Franks agreed to call the medical directors at the community health centers and at the hospital-based clinic for women. He also had started to list all of the family practice and OB/GYN physicians in the community. Doris agreed to contact the director of the now-closed Planned Parenthood clinic to negotiate the release of space, supplies, staff, and equipment to their public health offices if necessary. The Planned Parenthood Board of Directors and the chairperson of the county health council may also have some ideas. You said that you would call the state family planning program manager to see what resources they had available.

Within the week, a meeting was held with other health care providers in the community, the director of the Planned Parenthood clinic, the president of the Planned Parenthood Board of Directors, a representative for the county health council, and state public health officials. Shared values and common goals were developed that empowered the diverse group to focus on the problem-solving process and tackle this seemingly insurmountable problem.

> **Discuss the significance of community participation. Who is missing from this group?**

The next 30 days were hectic for you and your management team. It was a challenging situation, but it was time to plan a public health response as quickly as possible.

> **Give examples of each of the three core public health functions applied in this case. Discuss standardized approaches to planning community-oriented public health programs that you might apply here.**

Case Study #11

Homeless Health Care

―――――――――ぬ―――――――――

Learning Objectives

At the conclusion of this case, students will be able to

1. Describe the diversity of a homeless population
2. Identify sources of information about the homeless population
3. List the challenges encountered when planning a model of health care delivery for a homeless population
4. Discuss the evaluation component required in program planning

You are the program planner for a community health center in Birmingham, Alabama. The community health center in which you work is located in a low socioeconomic section of the city. Your health center was established in 1972 and provides primary care to a culturally diverse and indigent population. Many of the clients speak Spanish only.

As you review the federal register for the week, you come across an opportunity to apply for funding to provide primary care services to the homeless population. The executive director of the health center, who also read the request for proposals, assigns you the responsibility of writing the grant proposal. I don't know anything about the homeless population in Birmingham, you think. I have just 6 weeks to write this proposal. What should I do first?

In planning health services for a specific population, what do you need to know?

Some of the first questions that start to concern you are: How many homeless are in the city? Where are they? Who are they? What are their health problems? What kind of services do they need? Who else provides services to homeless people?

You decide to find out who comprises the homeless population nationally and in your city. To your surprise, not only single men but women, children, and families are homeless. Some are chronically homeless, and some are episodically homeless. Beyond the basic health care needs, many have mental and substance abuse problems, lack of life skills, poor family support, and are non-English speaking. A high number of veterans and elderly people also are homeless.

The homeless population has all of the usual health problems you would expect in the nonhomeless population, plus other problems resulting from their homeless lifestyle. Children need immunizations and nutritious food. The women need family planning and prenatal care. Sexually transmitted diseases, tuberculosis, AIDS, hepatitis, and other infectious diseases are common. Chronic disease management, exposure to extremes in weather, and insufficient rest are additional health issues. What about services for alcohol abuse, drug addiction, and mental illness?

How will you obtain this information about the homeless population? Who would you ask? What are the resources?

Collaboration and partnering with other health and social service agencies around community health issues are two principles to which your community health center subscribes. Successful collaboration and partnering rely on a common mission and shared goals among the collaborating agencies. Partnering brings in additional resources and reduces duplication and gaps in services. In the past, your agency has developed partnerships with other community health centers, social service centers, the local hospitals, a community mental health center, the school system, and the university.

What additional agencies could you contact for help in developing a comprehensive health care plan for the homeless in your city?

By contacting the human services department in your state, you learn that there are many private, not-for-profit, and volunteer organizations that provide food, temporary housing, used clothing and furniture, job skills, and detoxification services in your city. Some of the agencies require attendance at religious services prior to receiving a meal and a bed. Others have strict rules regarding the number of nights a person can use the facility in a month. To get a bed for the night, you must line up by 5:00 in the evening and be back out on the streets by 6:30 in the morning. Men and women, even if a family, are not allowed to stay in the same shelter. Some agencies require that you sign over your disability check to them to help pay for services. You have read in the paper about homeless men and women refusing to go into a shelter, even on inclement nights, fearing bodily injury. Others have died in fires while trying to keep warm in abandoned buildings.

What barriers to accessing health and social services confront the homeless? How can you overcome some of them in developing your plan for health care?

After assessing the needs of the homeless population and subpopulation groups in your city, you meet with the leaders of all of the agencies that provide services to the homeless. You want to ensure that your health care plan links with all of the other services provided. You learn that your city has six shelters for the homeless: one for battered women, one for women without children, one for mothers and children, and three for men. The location of the shelter for battered women is not advertised, but the other shelters are located within a

5-mile radius in the downtown area. Homeless people can go to one of three food banks for free food. In addition, many churches run soup kitchens.

Interviews with leaders in agencies providing services to the homeless reveal that many homeless do not seek health care until they are so sick or injured that they have to be transported to the hospital by ambulance. Lack of trust on the part of the homeless and judgmental care on the part of the health care providers are barriers to service. You also learn that competition for resources among the agencies providing services to the homeless interferes with their ability to collaborate.

Now that you have assessed the population and identified current resources for the homeless, you are ready to write a first draft of a health care plan for the homeless in your city.

> **Where will you provide care? Why? What disciplines do you need on your health care team? How will the homeless access health care? What are your goals and objectives for the plan? How will you know if your plan works?**

You decide to provide health care in the shelters because the homeless are familiar with these surroundings and the shelters have offered space. A mobile clinic is very expensive, requires a lot of maintenance, and requires access to parking and utility hookup. This is difficult in the busy downtown area. Instead of a mobile clinic, you propose a mobile health care team. The team will consist of a nurse, outreach worker, physician, nurse practitioner, social worker, and medical assistant/clerk. The outreach worker will visit the shelters and inform the homeless about the services. You will receive laboratory and pharmacy support from the parent community health center.

Essential to program development is the evaluation component. You decide to develop qualitative and quantitative methods of evaluation. You will measure structure, process, and outcome.

> **Define qualitative and quantitative, and structure, process, and outcome evaluation. Also, list three tools or methods you could use to evaluate the program.**

Case Study #12

Planning for School Health Services

Learning Objectives

At the conclusion of this case, students will be able to

1. Describe the special health care needs of middle school children
2. List the health care requirements for medically fragile children attending public school
3. List the steps necessary to collaboratively begin the planning process for a school-based health center in a conservative community

You are a school nurse for the Boone County School District. Boone County is a poor, rural county in southern Illinois. It is an unseasonably balmy day late in October. This is your first year as a school nurse in this district. Your scope of responsibility covers two elementary schools, one middle school, and one high school. Gazing out of your middle school office window at the vibrant fall colors, a

61

frown slowly creeps over your face. You have just finished reviewing the clinical records of all of the students in the middle school. These children have so many problems, you think to yourself.

What kind of health problems would you expect to occur in a population of middle school children?

You recall from your course in nursing school on health assessment that middle school children are preadolescent to early adolescence. They range in age between 10 and 14 years. Although children in this age group are basically healthy, their bodies and emotions are beginning to change. Accidents are the leading cause of death in this age group. Based on the children seeking your services over the past 6 weeks, you are also aware that these children are vulnerable to infectious respiratory and digestive diseases as well as accidents in the home, at play, and at school.

Having grown up in this community, you are aware of the poverty and social problems that occur. What other health problems occur in middle school children as a result of living in poverty in a rural community?

Your review of the children's clinical records and of your daily visit log reveals just what you expected. Many children had delays in physical, emotional, and behavioral development. Children came into your office hungry, dirty, and without proper clothing. Sometimes, you suspected child abuse. Many of the children listed "none" in the space on the student health information sheet that asked for the name of their family physician. Your frustration level increases as you say out loud, "How can I deal with all of these issues?"

You recently joined the State School Nurses Association. The major topic at the Association's last annual meeting was the challenges presented to school nurses on the mainstreaming of physically challenged children into the regular classroom. What demands could this action have on your role as a school nurse?

Glancing over at your paper-covered desk, a stack of clinical records greets your eyes. You pulled these records out during your review because they belong to the children with special health needs in the middle school. There are children who are diabetics and children with seizures. Some require frequent blood glucose checks and insulin injections. Some have severe asthma and require inhalation therapy. There are the Baldwin twins, born prematurely, and now severely retarded, unable to swallow and requiring tube feeding. The number of medications that must be administered during the school day is enormous! How can you manage the health of all of these children?

> **Having just assessed the health status of your student population, what are the appropriate health promotion and health maintenance strategies for children who are healthy as well as for these children with special health needs?**

You decide that you have two major roles as the school nurse in this middle school. One, for all children, you need to provide and support health promotion activities that increase their levels of health. Two, you need to provide an array of hands-on nursing skills to the children with special health care needs to maximize their potential. Both of these roles require prevention strategies. Children this age are rapidly changing physically and need adequate nutrition, rest, physical activity, and information about their safety. Interventions in these areas include providing health education activities that encourage the practice of healthy lifestyle behaviors. Screening is another valuable tool for identifying problems in health status even before symptoms appear. Some screening activities relevant to this school population include vision, hearing, scoliosis, hypertension, anemia, and dental. Health assessments are necessary to determine health risk behaviors and health histories.

Mulling over the nursing needs of the children with special health care needs in your middle school, you develop a list of skills you need to meet their needs. The list includes administering medications (orally and by injection), catheterization, administering oxygen and inhalants, fingersticks to check on blood sugar, and tube feedings.

> **As you look at your day planner and school rotation schedule, you recognize you cannot accomplish all of these roles by yourself. What is your next step?**

Although your school district superintendent and the community are supportive of you as the school nurse, they are very conservative. Remember your first parent-teacher meeting? High on the agenda was the mandate that there would be no reference to sexuality in the schools. To the community, school-based health services meant the distribution of condoms, birth control, and abortions. Many parents believe talking about sexuality, pregnancy, and sexually transmitted diseases makes it happen. Also, many parents are not happy about children with special health care needs attending their children's school. They feel it detracts from the educational environment.

You decide to get on the agenda of the next parent-teacher meeting and talk about the healthy middle school child and wellness. Your focus will be on healthy lifestyles and how health education can help the children develop positive behaviors. You will ask for volunteers to help with the clerical responsibilities of your job, freeing you to practice nursing.

> **Realizing that the school community is just one partner in this endeavor and that many parents do not attend the parent-teacher meetings, whom else would you contact?**

A mental assessment of your community identified a number of potential partners in this endeavor to keep school children healthy and to maximize the health of those who are physically, socially, and economically challenged. They include the public health department, the primary health care center, the county commissioners, the local family physician, the school of nursing at the community college, the chamber of commerce, and many, many others. Your job is to bring the message about school health issues to the community and obtain support to develop a school-based health center in the middle school.

Case Study #13

School Health/Border Issues

Learning Objectives

At the conclusion of this case, students will be able to

1. Discuss the concept *medically insured* and analyze its meaning in relation to farm workers
2. Understand the role of Medicaid
3. Discuss how changes in federal policy have given states the option of changing the rules of Medicaid and welfare

---

You are a school nurse in a small community close to the U.S.–Mexico border. You like the town very much, but lately, a number of concerns seem to be manifesting. The principal business in the area is agriculture, and your town is surrounded by fields of cotton, onions, and peppers. The people who do the work in the fields are, for the most part, migrant workers who follow the planting and harvesting season to the north and back again. Many "winter" in your community, and almost all are very poor. Most are legal workers, and many are citizens, but they often have difficulty with access to the health care system. Although many are eligible for Medicaid, the fact that they move from state to state makes it nearly impossible for them to have comprehensive coverage. The states vary in their eligibility requirements, and all require extensive documentation and paperwork in English. People feel intimidated by this system. For those who do apply for Medicaid, often, by the time the task is completed, they have moved on to another state. Women and children, as well as men, work in the fields, and the fragmented health care system results in little or no prenatal or pediatric care.

> What would be the results of this very hard fieldwork and little health care for mothers and children? Explore the issue of the medically uninsured in your group. Who provides care to the poor in very rural areas? Who pays? What are some of your state's regulations to be eligible for Medicaid, welfare, and food stamps? What is the WIC program? What are the implications of cutbacks in this program?

School started this week, and you discovered six children new to the school who do not seem to have their immunization records. Their parents, who are farmworkers, cannot remember whether they had measles vaccinations. Because the responsibility for immunization falls mainly on the schools, they cannot enter without the vaccinations. You know these children attend school very sporadically as they move from state to state with their parents. You want them to be able to attend school while they are in your community. You also appreciate that measles can be a serious disease, and that immunization is important. Without it, these children and others would be at risk.

Recently, there have been major changes in health care delivery in your town. Your state has initiated a Medicaid managed care system. As far as you understand it, a large, urban managed care organization (MCO) has a state contract to treat those on Medicaid. You know that several private physicians in town have contracted with the MCO to provide the care for this population. You are not sure which providers are connected to the MCO, and you do not know if the children are covered by Medicaid. You refer the parents of these children to the public health office to get the shots.

What is managed care? What is Medicaid managed care? Why has managed care become so popular? Perhaps you are enrolled in a managed care system. How does it work? Do you like it? How would this system work in rural areas?

You get a call from a friend at the public health office saying that the clinic is cutting back on its services and will no longer be issuing immunizations without documentation, that the recipients are not eligible for other services, such as Medicaid. He also tells you that the vaccines are no longer free. You hope that the parents get back in touch with you, because you have no idea where they are living. You are beginning to wonder where the uninsured people in your community will get primary care and what responsibility the school system has in this.

What role does public health have in your community? Why would this documentation be especially difficult for migrant workers? If, as in the case with measles, an outbreak can occur that can cause death to some who get it, whose responsibility is it to protect against the disease? What role in prevention and protection have the schools assumed? What role has the medical practice community assumed?

The parents of one of the children come to see you. They say they could not get the shots at the clinic. They want to know what to do now. You ask if they are eligible for Medicaid. They have been here only a few months, and they do not understand what this is. They have no documentation of income. They are legal workers from Mexico; they have been very poor, working at whatever jobs they could. They are staying with friends and have no money. They think their lives will improve here with the work in the fields, but they do not speak much English. How can they get their son into school?

Discuss the role of assessment, assurance, and policy development around the issues presented in this case. What public health policies and legislation has your state enacted recently? What are the trends in your state to provide health care for those who are uninsured?

Case Study #14

Health Promotion/Prevention of Diabetes Mellitus

Learning Objectives

At the conclusion of this case, students will be able to

1. Apply the steps in rational health program planning to a health problem
2. Understand the role of quantitative and qualitative data in needs assessment
3. Analyze and categorize individual and environmental determinants of disease
4. Write goals and objectives for a health program plan
5. Understand that health planning takes place in a social and political context

---

You have recently been employed by the Indian Health Service (IHS) as a health educator. You will be working with several tribes in a service unit in the Southwest. Your grandfather was a Cherokee Indian, but you know little about the Pueblo Indian tribes of the Southwest. You will be based in Santa Fe, New Mexico, in the IHS hospital, where you will share an office with other public health educators and nurses. You are meeting today with the health board for your service unit. You know that the eight members are representatives from each of the four tribes in the service unit, and that they act as advisors to the unit.

You have been studying the health problems of the Indian population in this area. You have learned that there are higher morbidity and mortality rates within this group for certain diseases and injuries. Mortality rates for the following are extremely high:

1. *Accidents:* In all age groups from 1 to 65, accidents are the leading cause of death for New Mexico Indians. The overall rate for this population is approximately four times the rate of the U.S. population, accounting for 20% of all Indian deaths in New Mexico each year. These accidents are predominantly motor vehicle-related (more than 50%).
2. *Suicide:* For young Indian males, the rates are two to three times the rates of the general U.S. population.
3. *Diabetes mellitus:* Mortality rates are five to six times higher than the general U.S. population for those 45 years and older.

You know that part of the mission of public health is to promote physical and mental health and prevent disease, injury, and disability. You want to hear what the health board members have to say about the problems in their communities.

The board meeting was very interesting. The largest tribe, Pueblo Bonito, wants to ask for more funding from IHS for next year's budget to finance a comprehensive diabetes project. They feel strongly that diabetes mellitus is a major health concern in their village, and they want it to become the number-one priority for the service unit. They ask you to help them substantiate the data and plan the project.

Summarize what is known so far. Look up diabetes mellitus in a reference book such as the *Merck Manual* and discuss the problem with your group. What is the most common type of diabetes? What is the problem? What are the most common

outcomes for patients who have it for a long period of time?
What information is needed now? Where can you go to get it?

You discover that IHS has epidemiologists in your area that monitor
the health status of the tribes. They provide you with the following
information from Pueblo Bonito:

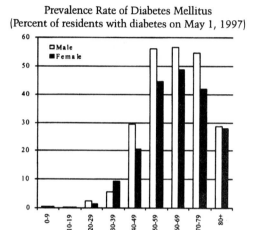

Prevalence Rate of Diabetes Mellitus
(Percent of residents with diabetes on May 1, 1997)

Based on 3-year resident active users of local IHS facilities

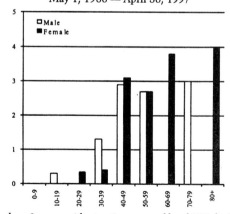

Incidence Rate of Diabetes Mellitus
(Percent of residents with onset of diabetes during 1 year)
May 1, 1966 — April 30, 1997

Based on 3-year resident active users of local IHS facilities

Figure 14.1. Incidence and Prevalence of Diabetes Mellitus, Pueblo Bonito, NM

What is the overall prevalence of diabetes in the Pueblo? What
else can be ascertained from the data presented? You know that
community involvement is vital to any health program planning.
What are the next steps?

You have a long discussion with your office mates, who have been
IHS employees for a long time. There are an estimated 9 million people with diabetes in the United States. Less than 10% are insulin-
dependent, known as Type I. Type II, non-insulin-dependent diabetes,
is characterized by a tissue insensitivity to insulin that is being
normally produced. You learn that diabetes patients share a similar
profile. They are nearly all overweight, they have sedentary lifestyles,
and their diet is high in calories and fat. Diabetes also seems to run
in families. Exercise and diet control can have an effect on disease
management and onset. The chronic complications from the disease
can include cataracts, glaucoma, end-stage renal disease, gangrene,
heart disease, and amputations. The age of onset in your service unit
for the disease is dropping; people are being diagnosed with the disease
at a younger age. The social conditions in Pueblo Bonito include high
rates of unemployment and poverty. The relative isolation of the
Pueblo necessitates long driving to get to a large town.

What are some of the determinants for diabetes? Be sure to
include host and environmental factors. Which determinants
can be addressed in a health program? Organize the
determinants into those that are best addressed in a medical
setting and those that belong in a public health setting. Are
some of the determinants amenable to change? Can there be a
role for prevention in diabetes? List some prevention strategies
under the primary, secondary, and tertiary prevention categories.

You are going to prepare a health program plan. You understand the
complexity of the disease and the difficulties that accompany an
intervention. You want to find out what the communities think about
the disease and the consequences. You want the community involved
in the planning process.

What do you do now? How can you gather both quantitative
and qualitative data to support need? How can you get the

communities involved? Keep them involved? What do you want to do first?

You have the needs assessment data to support the enormity of the problem. You are ready to begin planning the intervention. Select a recorder for your group to write the draft plan. Begin with an overall goal. Create several objectives to support the goal. Use the determinants you selected earlier to guide your plan. Include objectives in clinical management as well as objectives for prevention. Use the prevention strategies you listed above to make action steps to support your objectives. Remember to make your objectives very clear. They should say who is doing what and when. At this point, your plan should contain a statement of need, a program goal, objectives, action steps, an approximate time frame, and the people and organizations responsible for the program.

The next case, Case Study #15, will involve the evaluation of the program.

Case Study #15

Health Promotion Program Evaluation

Learning Objective

At the conclusion of this case, students will be able to

1. Develop an evaluation protocol for a health program plan that includes process, program impact, and health outcome evaluation components

This case study will use the information developed in Case Study #14. You and your colleagues at the IHS service unit have prepared a draft health program plan to address diabetes mellitus in Pueblo Bonito. Today, you are all meeting to discuss how the evaluation component will be developed for the plan. You realize that evaluation is somewhat difficult to understand and incorporate into programs, and you want to know more about it. The meeting begins with a question about what evaluation really means.

> What is meant by evaluation? Why bother? Make a list of
> several reasons why evaluation should take place. What kind of
> information do you want? How might this information benefit
> the program?

There are lots of questions about the evaluation process. Administrators, clinical providers, and public health practitioners such as yourself are attending the meeting. Everyone seems to have a different idea about what should be included. You realize that there are many parts to the program that need to be assessed.

> How do you decide the standards for evaluation? What are the
> main types of evaluation? Discuss the variety of items that could
> be evaluated in your diabetes project. Do they all fit into the
> same category? Group these items into similar types of
> evaluation or categories.

Your group analyzes the program objectives and realizes that those that are written with clear baseline data are easier to evaluate. Some of the objectives relate to the administrative part of the program, some are concerned with prevention, and some relate to the improved clinical management of diabetes. A change in the incidence of the disease seems to be measureable but only after a considerable length of time has passed. Other items can be measured very quickly.

> Analyze your goal(s) for your project. How will this goal be
> evaluated? Who will be responsible for doing the evaluation, and
> where will the data come from? How long will it take to see
> whether the program might have made a difference? How will
> you know if it is the program that made the difference? You have
> calculated the prevalence of diabetes in Pueblo Bonito. Should
> this number be used for a standard? How? Have you set a
> number that will indicate program success? Where would that
> number come from? What is reasonable to attain?

The discussion evolves into consideration of evaluation design. How to know whether the intervention worked and, if there is success, how to know whether it was actually due to the intervention are the overriding questions.

> **What are some basic evaluation designs? How could you improve the knowledge of whether or not the intervention worked? How could you know more about whether or not the success was due to the intervention?**

To improve the quality of the evaluation information, you decide on a "comparison" group design.

> **What does this mean? How could this be done in your service unit?**

It is clear that much remains to be done to complete the health program plan. You set up another meeting to review the current objectives and consider the issues in developing the mechanisms for program evaluation.

> **Using the objectives you developed in Case Study #14, analyze whether they do what you really want to do in the program. Can they be measured? How would they be measured? What instruments are needed? Will weight loss be measured? Where will it be done? What about reliability and validity? If information is self-reported, what are the problems? Is exercise a component of the intervention? How will the levels of exercise be measured? Will blood sugar levels be taken periodically? Where? Who will do this? Does the objective clearly state the intent?**

> **Outline an evaluation protocol that includes study design and methods for evaluating your program goal and objectives. What about the baseline data? Who will collect it? Where? What about the comparison group? Do you need to create instruments and pretest? Include reliability and validity assessments? Will you use questionnaires? Interviews? Who will collect the information? Do they have the time and training to do this?**

About the Authors

Jo Fairbanks, PhD, is currently teaching in the Master's in Public Health degree program at the University of New Mexico School of Medicine. In addition to extensive classroom experience, she has also spent many years in public health practice. She uses problem-based learning in all of her classes. Dr. Fairbanks is a co-author of *The Public Health Primer* (1998).

Judith Candelaria, MSN, RN, is the chief of the Chronic Disease Prevention & Control Bureau in the New Mexico Department of Health. She also teaches part-time in the nursing program at the University of Phoenix, New Mexico campus. She has 20 years of experience in community and public health practice settings in both staff and management roles.

The case studies in *Case Studies in Community Health* are drawn from the authors' experiences.